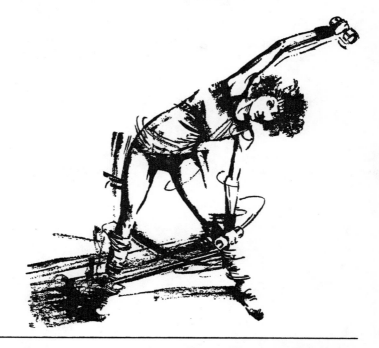

FIRMING UP YOUR FLABBY FAITH

Firming Up
YOUR
FLABBY FAITH

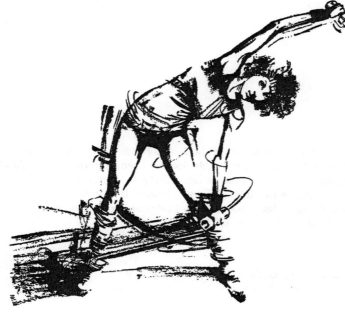

VICKI LAKE

VICTOR BOOKS®
A DIVISION OF SCRIPTURE PRESS PUBLICATIONS INC.
USA CANADA ENGLAND

Recommended Dewey Decimal Classification: 227.91
Suggested Subject Heading: BIBLE, N.T., EPISTLES—JAMES

Library of Congress Card Catalog Number: 90-60255
ISBN: 0-89693-783-6

1 2 3 4 5 6 7 8 9 10 Printing/Year 94 93 92 91 90

VICTOR BOOKS
A division of SP Publications, Inc.
Wheaton, Illinois 60187

CONTENTS

23506

We are living in the era of the "fitness craze." One cannot read a newspaper or magazine without being conscious of the many references to the importance of being physically fit. Walk through a store only to see racks of sweat suits and workout gear beautifully displayed. *USA Today* newspaper recently carried a full-page ad featuring Nike shoes. Browse through a bookstore, even a Christian bookstore, and find books, sometimes best-sellers, that deal with being physically fit. In fact, I have one on my bookshelf above my typewriter that is titled *The Aerobics Program for Total Well-Being*. Ironically, right beside it is *Let's Make a Memory*. For some, exercising is definitely making a memory!

Why all the fuss over fitness? The benefits of exercise are many and I would not make light of exercise. It takes far more than putting on a sweat suit or donning aerobic exercise shoes. But I am also reminded of Paul's words to Timothy: Train yourself to be godly. For physical training is of some value, but godliness has value for all things, holding promise for both the present life and life to come" (1 Timothy 4:7-8).

What if as much emphasis were given to spiritual fitness as physical fitness? Would it make a difference? James has much to say regarding spiritual fitness and you definitely will be challenged during your study of this book.

If you are using this book for personal study only, then you will want to complete each chapter that follows. If you plan to use the book for group study as well, you will want to use the Leader's Guide at the end of the book.

Each chapter is divided into several sections. Stretching Your Spiritual Muscles will enable you to do an inductive study of James. You will want to read thoroughly and thoughtfully the Scripture passages given and pray for wisdom as you answer the questions. Exercising Your Spiritual Muscles, a narrative section, will explain and enlarge some spiritual concepts introduced in the first section. Disciplining for Daily Exercise is a journaling section intended to help you begin or maintain the daily disciplines of reading, applying, and memorizing God's Word.

Hang in there as you begin to stretch, exercise, and flex your spiritual muscles in order to firm up your flabby faith.

SPIRITUAL FITNESS INVENTORY

1. Am I becoming "bitter" or "better" as a result of the "trying" exercises in my life?
2. Am I asking for God's wisdom instead of relying on my own in the midst of the "trying" exercises?
3. Is there anything in my life which has control of me instead of my controlling it?
4. Do I have God's divine nature within me as a result of making Him my personal Saviour and Lord? Am I realizing God's divine nature within me to help me with the "tempting" enticements?
5. When receiving God's Word,
    Am I "swift to hear"?
    Am I "slow to speak"?
    Am I "slow to wrath"?
    Am I "cleansed"?
6. Do I look intently into the mirror of God's Word and not do anything about my spiritual condition?
7. Do I show favoritism to others?
8. Do I constantly look to Jesus as the example in relationships with all people?
9. Am I "tripping over" or "tying up" my tongue?
10. Have I allowed the Lord to tie my tongue with the "heart strings" of which He has control?
11. When someone else's tongue is out of control, do I
    avoid the flame?
    fan the flame?
    ask for a firefighter's wisdom to control the flame?
    douse the flame?
    pray about the burns?
12. Am I genuinely sorrowful and repentant for the sins I've committed?
13. Have I humbled myself and submitted to God's control over my life? Have I stepped into God's "whirlpool of submission"?
14. Am I more concerned with the world's riches than I am with spiritual richness?
15. Am I prepared for the Lord's return? Am I prayerful? Am I patient? Am I on patrol? Watchful?

16. Am I sincerely and humbly seeking to restore others to spiritual health?

If after taking the Spiritual Fitness Inventory, you realize that there are areas in your life that need shaping up, take a few moments in prayer to ask for the Lord's wisdom and strength to help you in these areas. Those few moments spent with Him can be the best investment you can ever make toward your becoming spiritually fit.

Don't put away this Spiritual Fitness Inventory never to take it again. Place it in your Bible or notebook to constantly check yourself. I find that there are always new areas in my life which I need to commit to the best Fitness Expert of all—the Lord.

CHAPTER ONE

THE TRYING

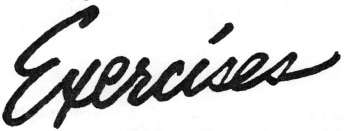

STRETCHING YOUR
❧ SPIRITUAL MUSCLES ❧

Read James 1:1-12.
1. What does James 1:2 tell us to do when we face trials? How do the following passages tell us to regard our trials?
   Job 13:15   2 Corinthians 4:18
   Job 23:10-12   2 Thessalonians 1:4-5
   Psalm 66:10   1 Peter 1:7

2. What should be the end result of our trials? Describe the actions/attitudes of a person who has become bitter instead of better as a result of trials.

How do you respond to a bitter person?

How do you respond to someone who has triumphed in trials? Identify some people who have been victors instead of victims in the trials of life.

3. What do you think *perfection* (NASB) means in verses 3-4? In what ways could you be perfect according to these verses?

4. What are we to ask for that will help us in our trials? (vv. 5-6) How are we to ask? How does God give?

5. Describe God's wisdom according to Proverbs 3:13-21 and 8:1-21.

   What qualities of wisdom do you especially desire?

6. What comfort do you find in Romans 8:28? Record a time in your life when God took a seemingly bad situation and made something beautiful out of it.

7. What will those who persevere under trials receive?

8. Name some things in this past year that were specific trials in your life. How did you respond to them?

What are you like today as a result of those trials? Bitter or better? Victim or victor?

Can you say with Job in Job 32:10, "I shall come forth as gold"? If you are bitter, claim 1 John 1:9 and Proverbs 3:5-6.

EXERCISING YOUR
🦾 SPIRITUAL MUSCLES 🦾

A friend once gave me a *Cathy* poster which I strategically placed by my jogging trampoline. As Cathy is jogging, she reminds herself, "This is very healthy. This is very healthy. This is very healthy . . ."

Like Cathy, I have to constantly remind myself that exercise is healthy. I don't like exercise. As a matter of fact, I think only a few people's faces are filled with exhilaration when exercising. However, I do enjoy the benefits of exercise. My family says I look all-around healthier when I'm regularly exercising. Now, isn't that a kind way to recognize the firmed-up flab?

There are other benefits, as well. The muscles become better toned, the heart strengthened, endurance increased, and stress relieved. I just have to keep reminding myself of the end results while struggling through the pain and sweat.

Just as muscles grow through exercise, faith grows through testing. I don't like the trials in this life that come my way. Who does? I've never heard anyone say, "Oh, I just love pain!" or "Aren't troubles wonderful?" Yet, James in his epistle tells us that we can triumph in the trying exercises of this life.

James emphasizes the inevitability of the trying exercises while giving four imperatives to triumphing. James 1:2 says not "if" but "when" you face trials. We don't have a choice. Pain and suffering are part and parcel of our planet.

The Greek word for trials is *perirasmos* which draws the word picture of a refining fire where the dross is removed and the gold refined. If gold had feelings and could talk, it might shout from the fire amidst the flames of pain, "Just wait and see. I shall come forth as gold." It isn't easy to recognize beauty in brokenness, yet that is exactly the first imperative James gives when he writes, "Consider it pure joy" (1:2). In other words, we are to evaluate our trials in light of what God can do.

Sounds crazy, but perhaps you've seen beauty in brokenness. I have.

We took my friend and her children with us on vacation to the beach just a few weeks after her husband told her he was divorcing her and leaving her with the children. With permission, I share words I penned one day after she and I had sat in the surf.

> Silently we sat.
> Loudly the surf of the sea tumbled into foam.
> The sand, wedged between our toes, slowly trickled away
> Leaving a place of emptiness.
>
> Silently we cried.
> Loudly the memories of the past weeks crashed into thoughts.
> Her husband, confused and wayward, quickly wandered away
> Leaving a family of heartaches.
>
> Silently I tried.
> Gradually my eyes of tears turned toward the sand.
> The shells, broken and worn, slowly piled ashore
> Comprising a formation of beauty.
>
> Softly I spoke,
> "There can be beauty in brokenness."
>
> Silently we prayed.

God answered prayer and in the midst of a seemingly impossible situation, the husband returned to an even more beautiful wife because through it all, she had learned to totally trust God.

Secondly, James tells us to know that the testing of our faith works patience and patience produces perfection. I've always enjoyed the thought of perfection. So many of us think that perfection is unattainable. However, the perfection (*telios*) in James means that an object is being used for what it was intended.

Last summer while my husband was on a six-week sabbatical, some dear members of our church made their beach condominium available to us. As we left, they said we'd especially enjoy the bicycles. The condo was absolutely wonderful, but the bikes were a little less desirable. Old, rusty, old, tarnished, old, wobbly . . . Did I say old? In fact, our eleven-year-old daughter insisted that there was only one of the four she would even consider riding. But before the week was over, we had come to realize just how perfect (*telios*) those bicycles were. They provided transportation to the beach and around the plantation. We often laughed as we stopped to retrack one of the chains. Those old bikes brought us closer as a family.

As I've reflected on the "perfect" bicycles, I've thought about how God uses people who are perfectly fulfilling their purpose in order to bring praise to Him. Some are broken, some are bruised, and some are even struggling, yet God uses them. I've met many missionaries in less-than-perfect settings with less-than-perfect personalities that God is perfectly using to impact others.

The third imperative for triumphing in trying exercises is "Let patience have her perfect work in you" (1:4, KJV). In other words, we are to let go and let God. It is a process of releasing which I'll admit isn't always easy. Sometimes God doesn't move as fast as we think He should, but I've come to realize that His timing is always perfect.

We have a beloved "adopted" daughter of missionary parents who came to live in our home for approximately a year after she became very angry over the death of a close friend and quit college. We grew to love her unconditionally in her agony and anger. She and I spent much time talking over her perplexities and problems. I often prayed for patience as I released her to the Lord and His perfect timing. In due time, she too released her frustrations to Him and is one of the most radiant, vibrant Christians I know. She is happily married to a young man whose ministry reaches into several countries of the world.

The last imperative is found in James 1:5-6. We are to ask for wisdom realizing that God gives generously to all who ask without doubting. God will help us make discerning decisions in difficult situations. When is the last time you asked for His wisdom?

We have looked at the inevitability of the trying exercises, their influence, and the imperatives to triumph. James then tells us the incentive: "Blessed is the man who perseveres under trial, because when he has stood the test, he will receive the crown of life that God has promised to those who love him" (1:12).

Do you know someone who has already received the crown? Our church most recently watched a thirty-two year old lady named Nancy Byers slip into eternity to receive her crown. I've never seen anyone suffer more victoriously as cancer riddled her body over a period of two years. Nancy taught us how to be better not bitter, a victor not a victim in trials. In the midst of her horrendous pain, she told a friend one day, "I don't have any bad days. Some days are just better than others."

What a joy to realize that when the trying exercises of this life are over and we stand before the King of kings, He will place a "crown of victory" of His Divine approval on our heads. Have you allowed Him to make you victor instead of victim in the trying exercises of your life?

DISCIPLINING FOR
❧ DAILY EXERCISE ❧

To firm up your flabby faith you must understand the importance of daily exercising in God's Word. This section will help you read from God's Word each day. In the space provided, write some ways that you can apply the truth you've discovered. You will also be given a portion of Scripture to memorize on the first day of each week. Repeat the verse each day for the remainder of the week. Entrusting God's Word to memory will keep your faith firm and strong.

SUNDAY: Approaching God's Word: 1 Peter 5:10
                Applying God's Word:

Memorizing God's Word: Romans 8:28

MONDAY: Approaching God's Word: 1 Corinthians 2:9-10
                Applying God's Word:

TUESDAY: Approaching God's Word: Romans 8:37-39
                Applying God's Word:

WEDNESDAY: Approaching God's Word: John 16:33
                Applying God's Word:

18

THURSDAY: Approaching God's Word: 2 Corinthians 12:7-10
                  Applying God's Word:

FRIDAY: Approaching God's Word: Hebrews 12:11
                  Applying God's Word:

SATURDAY: Approaching God's Word: Romans 5:3-5
                  Applying God's Word:

CHAPTER TWO

THE TEMPTING

Enticements

STRETCHING YOUR
❧ SPIRITUAL MUSCLES ❧

Read James 1:13-18.

1. What does James 1:13-16 say about the process of temptation?

Describe a time when you experienced the process in your own life?

2. Read 1 John 2:15-17 and describe lust.

3. Give the views given in James 1:13-15 concerning the source of temptation.

Why would a person blame God for sending temptation his or her way?

What is the real cause of temptation? Review Mark 7:20-23 and Romans 7:14-18.

4. What are the consequences of sin? (Romans 7:5)

5. What is comforting to you regarding the character of God as described in James 1:17?

How do the following scriptures describe God?

Numbers 14:17-19

1 Samuel 15:29

Psalm 3

John 3:16

2 Thessalonians 3:5

2 Peter 3:8-9

6. Describe God's gifts to us according to James 1:18.

Why are these gifts important, especially in overcoming temptation?

Relate a specific time when these gifts helped you.

7. Why are you tempted? Read also 1 Peter 5:7-10. With what are you most easily tempted?

When and where are you most easily tempted?

Can you do anything about the temptation?

8. What was Jesus' weapon against Satan's temptations in Matthew 4:1-11?

9. How can the advice given in Colossians 3:1-3, 5 help us in overcoming temptations?

EXERCISING YOUR
❧ *SPIRITUAL MUSCLES* ❧

I've often wondered if fattening foods have special communication systems that link directly to our brains. Imagine a delectable, delicious piece of chocolate pie calling, "Come and eat. I have a wonderful taste, and you won't be sorry." Even when we are dieting to trim away the excess and doing our best to be physically fit, we may struggle with the temptations to savor or gorge. In the same way, though we often know what it takes to be spiritually fit, the temptations remain. James 1:13-18 delineates not only the process of temptation but also the protection against temptation.

First of all, James mentions the role of our own desires in the process of temptation. God gives us desires to be enjoyed, but when *enjoyment yields to engrossment*, we quickly fall into dangerous territory. Our desires are much like the steam in a boiler which is necessary to make the engine work, but when the steam gets out of control, disaster prevails. In 1 John 2:15-17, lust, materialism, and pride are listed as examples of evil desires. "The world and its desires pass away, but the man who does the will of God lives forever" (2:17). We must not let our enjoyments become engrossments.

The next step in the process involves Satan and his role. When I taught high school English, a student named Michael would often entertain our class with his antics. However, there were times when his antics would adversely affect the classroom and I would need to discipline him. His pat answer would be, "But, Mrs. Lake, the devil made me do it." To which I would quickly reply, "Michael, the devil tempts. You yield. The devil dangles the bait. You bite."

The devil knows precisely which bait to use on each of us. His tackle box must be the biggest one in the world. The lure he uses on one line may be entirely different than the one he uses on another. He aims to trap and his *enticement yields to entrapment* if we yield. It is difficult not to become entrapped in a society that shouts, "Do your own thing. If it feels good, do it. You are a god to yourself. Take care of yourself first. How can it be wrong when it feels so right?"

First John 2:14 describes young men who are strong and overcome the evil one as men in whom the Word of God lives. Christ set the example in Matthew 4 as He used Scripture to combat Satan's temptations. The Word of God must be our best defense in not becoming entrapped by his enticements. In the spiritual armor described in Ephesians 6, it is the only piece used both offensively and defensively.

The last step of the process is really not a step but a falling down—a fall into *endless destruction* and death. "Then, after desire has conceived, it gives birth to sin; and sin, when it is full-grown, gives birth to death" (James 1:15). What an awful, awesome thought to realize that sin spawns death. The word picture is that of giving birth to an animal. In actuality, when we follow the process of temptation, we are becoming like animals who are mastered by their desires rather than mastering their desires. We've all witnessed people hopelessly lost in their sins and mastered by their desires.

James doesn't leave us with the bait dangling in front of us. He gives us protection against temptation in 1:15-18. He forces us to *consider God's judgment of death.* That in itself should keep us from habitually sinning. We should also *consider God's goodness.* I've always liked the Hallmark commercials that say, "When you care enough to send the very best." When I see or hear that slogan, I think of the fact that God cared enough to send the very best—His precious Son to sacrifice Himself on the Cross for my sins. James 1:17 reminds us that every good and perfect gift comes from the Father above who, as the Living Bible states, is the Creator of all light, and shines forever without change or shadow. The reminder of His contributions and constancy alone can keep me constant in my own spiritual fitness.

But He gives us more. He gives us His Word and wants to give us spiritual birth and new life through Jesus Christ, the Word that became flesh and dwelt among us. It is the Bible that points to the Living Word, Jesus. It is also the Bible that encourages us on how to be spiritually fit. I have often quoted God's Word in times of discouragement and temptation. I especially love 2 Timothy 1:7 when tempted to be engrossed with fear: "For God did not give us a spirit of timidity, but a spirit of power, of love and of self-discipline."

I suffer with Chronic Epstein-Barr Virus Syndrome and it is God's Word that has been the best medicine when doctors offer no hope. Just yesterday Psalm 94:19 was the verse that helped me through a difficult day. "Lord, when doubts fill my mind, when my heart is in turmoil, quiet me and give me renewed hope and cheer."

As James 1:18 calls these early Christians "firstfruits," I realize that when I have put my faith and trust in Jesus Christ, I am His offspring. I have His power within to overcome enticements by Satan. I *consider God's divine nature within me.*

A few years ago, my younger daughter was reciting her memory verse. I wasn't paying too much attention until my older daughter snickered and pointed to her sister. As I listened I heard a sweet, little voice saying, "This is my beloved Son in whom I am well-done." As I thought of her version of Matthew 17:5, it became difficult for me to correct her words from "well-done" to "well pleased" because in Jesus we are "well-done." He has made available every capacity to be spiritually fit, to not yield to temptation. Philippians 2:13 reminds us that "it is God who works in you to will and to act according to His good purpose."

DISCIPLINING FOR
🎗 DAILY EXERCISE 🎗

Use this section to help you read from God's Word each day. Repeat the memory verse each day for the remainder of the week. Remember, entrusting God's Word to memory will keep your faith firm and strong.

SUNDAY: Approaching God's Word: 1 Corinthians 10:12-13
                              Applying God's Word:

Memorizing God's Word: 1 Corinthians 10:13

MONDAY: Approaching God's Word: Proverbs 1:10; 4:14
                              Applying God's Word:

TUESDAY: Approaching God's Word: Romans 6:13
                              Applying God's Word:

WEDNESDAY: Approaching God's Word: Ephesians 6:11, 13
                              Applying God's Word:

THURSDAY: Approaching God's Word: 1 John 4:4; James 4:7
                       Applying God's Word:

FRIDAY: Approaching God's Word: Hebrews 2:18; 2 Peter 2:9
                       Applying God's Word:

SATURDAY: Approaching God's Word: Revelation 3:10
                       Applying God's Word:

CHAPTER THREE

THE FAITH
Workout

STRETCHING YOUR
❧ SPIRITUAL MUSCLES ❧

Read James 1:19-27.
1. How should we prepare ourselves for the receiving of God's Word?

2. What do the following scriptures have to say regarding listening?

    1 Samuel 3:9

    1 Kings 19:11-13

    Psalm 46:10

    Proverbs 1:5

    Proverbs 12:15

    Proverbs 18:13

    Ecclesiastes 5:1-3

John 10:27

How have you been listening to God lately?

3. According to James 1:21, of what are we to rid ourselves?

Explain this verse in light of Ephesians 4:22 and Colossians 3:5-10.

Are there things of which you need to rid yourself?

4. With what attitude are we to receive the Word of God?

5. What does the implanted Word of God do in our lives? See also John 17:17; Romans 1:16; and 1 Corinthians 1:18.

6. According to Matthew 13:19-22, what are the different ways Jesus said the Word of God can be received?

Which type of soil best describes your spiritual receptivity?

7. To what does James compare the Word of God in James 1:22-25?

How often do you make changes in your appearance each day after looking at a mirror?

How often do you make changes as a result of looking into God's Word?

8. Why does James call the Word of God the "perfect law that gives freedom"? (1:25)

How do the following Scriptures further explain?

John 8:31-32, 34

Romans 8:2

Psalm 119:45

Read James 2:14-26.
9. Describe Abraham's faith.

Describe Rahab's faith.

10. What should be evidence of our faith?

What is evidence of your faith? If someone were trying you for your faith, would there be enough evidence to convict you?

EXERCISING YOUR
&c SPIRITUAL MUSCLES &c

Dwight L. Moody was once quoted as saying, "Every Bible should be bound in shoe leather." When I first heard the quote in my younger days, I laughed, not realizing the significance of his words. I thought he meant that shoe leather would probably be more durable and the Bible would last longer. As I've seen faith worked out in my life and others' lives, I know what he meant. God's Word becomes so much more alive and real when we see its influence and power worked out in the lives of individuals. James has much to say about faith being worked out in a Christian's life. Faith becomes flabby if it is not exercised.

I have always enjoyed gardening. Every step of the process excites me, especially the preparation of the soil. I get itchy fingers every spring to dig in the dirt. It must be a reversion to childhood sandbox days. However, I am most happy if I can break up the clumps, pull the weeds, disengage the stones, and till the ground to ready the soil for the seeds. James 1:19-21 describes the process of *readying the soil*, our hearts, for the receiving of the seed of God's Word.

In order to ready our hearts, we must, first of all, *close our mouths*—"be swift to hear." I often enjoy sitting as still as possible and listening to sounds around me. Right now, I can hear children playing, an airplane flying, all kinds of birds singing, the fish tank bubbling, the refrigerator motor humming, and the pen writing. Isn't it great that God gave us two ears and one mouth so we could hear twice as much as we speak? But do we?

Secondly, we must *control our speech*—"be slow to speak." How often do we speak before truly listening? "He who answers before listening— that is his folly and shame" (Proverbs 18:13). "He who holds his tongue is wise" (Proverbs 10:19). James 1:26 tells us to keep a tight rein on our tongues.

Thirdly, we must *check our tempers*—"be slow to wrath." I would liken anger in our lives to rocks in the soil that prohibit growth. James 1:20

indicates "anger does not bring about the righteous life that God desires."

Lastly, we should *cleanse our lives*—"get rid of all moral filth and the evil that is so prevalent." I find it interesting that the root of the Greek word for filth is *rupos* which means wax in the ear. The filth keeps us from hearing God's Word as we should. The Greek for "the evil that is so prevalent" represents overgrown weeds and tangled undergrowth. How relevant that just as the weeds must be pulled to allow growth in the soil, the weeds of evil must be pulled from our lives in order to allow spiritual growth from the planting of God's Word. Are there any overgrown weeds which need to be pulled from our gardens?

The next step after readying the soil is the *receiving of the seed*, God's Word. James even tells us that we should humbly receive the Word. When we read or listen to God's Word, we should have teachable attitudes.

When I approach God's Word each day during my quiet time, I pray, "Lord, I come empty today. What do you want to teach me from your Word." I then look for peace. Peace for me is spelled as follows: **P**—Promises to claim; **E**—Examples to follow or not follow; **A**—Attitudes to possess or not possess; **C**—Commands to obey; **E**—Enlargement of my thoughts of God. God has been so faithful to teach me and give me peace from His Word.

When I approach His Word, I also pray, "Lord, help me make changes in my life that You show me are necessary for spiritual progress." How many times have we looked in a mirror today? Have we made any changes in our appearances as a result? I've often thought what we'd all look like if we were minus the mirrors. It could be very interesting as well as amusing. James states that if we approach God's Word without applying its message to our lives, we are like someone who looks in a mirror, sees something wrong, and walks away without making the necessary adjustments.

My neighbors must laugh at me as I walk around our yard each spring. I laughingly call myself the "Pre-Spring Peeker" because I get so excited over the first signs of growth. One day my daughters had a silent wager that I wouldn't drive them to the gymnastic lesson without pointing out some of the beautiful signs of spring. Needless to say, they chuckled when I pointed out some tulips a few blocks into our journey. I can't help it! I get excited when I see the results of planting. I get more excited, however, when I see Christians who have readied their hearts for receiving God's Word and are *responding with the fruit*. They are doing what God's Word says. James 1:22 says "Do not merely listen to the Word, and so deceive yourselves. Do what it says." If the love of God is within us, it should overflow into the lives of others. First John

3:16-18 shows how Christ set the example of love by laying down His life. We, likewise, should be willing to lay down our lives for others. If we are selfish when someone is in need, how can the love of God be within? We must love not only with our words but also with our actions.

James gives a warning for unprepared and unfruitful soil. He states that "faith by itself, if it is not accompanied by action, is dead" (2:17). It would be obvious to me that if a seed or plant showed no signs of growth after being planted, that it was dead.

Churches are filled with people who readily declare their faith by quoting: "For it is by grace you have been saved, through faith—and this not from yourselves, it is the gift of God—not by works, so that no one can boast" (Ephesians 2:8-9). But those same people hesitantly confirm that faith with their deeds. They forget to quote the following verse: "For we are God's workmanship, created in Christ Jesus to do good works, which God prepared in advance for us to do" (2:10).

A strenuous physical workout is not always easy, just as it isn't always easy to show forth our Christianity by actions. Yet, the results are beneficial and readily show the fruits of our labor.

DISCIPLINING FOR
🦶 DAILY EXERCISE 🦶

SUNDAY: Approaching God's Word: Psalm 1:1-3
                Applying God's Word:

                Memorizing God's Word: Ephesians 2:10

MONDAY: Approaching God's Word: Jeremiah 17:5-8
                Applying God's Word:

TUESDAY: Approaching God's Word: Ephesians 4:13-16
                Applying God's Word:

WEDNESDAY: Approaching God's Word: Psalm 139:23-24
                Applying God's Word:

THURSDAY: Approaching God's Word: Matthew 5:16
                Applying God's Word:

FRIDAY: Approaching God's Word: Matthew 25:31-40
                           Applying God's Word:

SATURDAY: Approaching God's Word: Joshua 1:8-9
                           Applying God's Word:

CHAPTER FOUR

THE ONLY

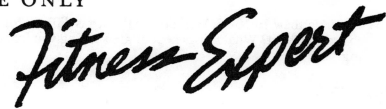

STRETCHING YOUR
🎗 SPIRITUAL MUSCLES 🎗

Read James 2:1-13.
1. According to 2:1 what two things are incompatible?

2. What example of favoritism does James give in 2:2-3?

Why do you think the favoritism happened?

How can favoritism manifest itself in churches today?

3. What belongs to the poor who love Christ?

Read Matthew 19:16-26. Why do you think it is difficult for the rich to accept Christ? What things kept or are keeping you from accepting Christ?

4. Read the following passages, noticing how Jesus was impartial in His relationships with people.

Matthew 11:4-5

Luke 4:18-19

John 4:7-10

5. What is the royal law that is reiterated in James 2:8?

If the royal law were kept, do you think the Ten Commandments would be necessary? Why or why not?

6. According to Luke 10:25-37 who is our neighbor?

According to Matthew 25:35-36 to whom are we really ministering when we reach out to others?

7. How is showing favoritism viewed in James 2:9?

Who is guilty of breaking the whole law?

8. Who will be judged mercilessly according to James 2:13?

Read Romans 14:10-13. Who will be the only spiritual fitness expert?

Read Matthew 7:1-5. What happens when we begin to judge others?

9. Have you ever been guilty of being a respecter of persons in any of your relationships? Are you prejudiced? If so, you can ask for forgiveness and begin now to love as Christ loves.

10. Is there someone you are having difficulty loving? What help can you find in Matthew 5:43-48?

EXERCISING YOUR
🍂 SPIRITUAL MUSCLES 🍂

No way, I thought as I jealously watched the teens I had chaperoned disperse into the little, remote Haitian village to share their witness of Christ. I turned around to view all the sick people packed onto the wooden benches in the crudely built, two-room church. I had not desired to stay and help in the medical clinic after the service. However, Linda, the nurse in charge, had asked me to help her. I had already decided that dispensing pills was the least threatening job, yet, to my dismay she had decided that cleaning and bandaging sores and wounds was a job I could handle. It was an ugly job! However, through that job the Lord squelched my pride and showed me His love for all kinds of people.

In the little side room with a dirt floor, I met my first patient, a small, quiet lady with big sad eyes and an open ulcerated sore from her foot to her knee. I swallowed quickly, prayed fervently, and cleaned carefully. *Why me, God,* I protested inside. When I finished the disgusting job, she stood up and suddenly threw her arms around me. I felt as if I'd been hugged by God. Tears trickled down both our cheeks. There are moments in our lives when we feel His permeating presence, and, for me, that was one. I knew God loved her in her poverty just as much as He loved me in my pride. Yet, my pride could be and was surrendered at that moment. Her poverty was unaltered.

James 2:1-13 has much to say regarding favoritism. We will look at the command, the condition of the church, the cause, and the cure.

James 2:1 commands that we are not to show favoritism: "Don't be a respecter of persons." Faith in Christ and partiality are incompatible. In the Greek the words for *favoritism* mean to receive by face. It was necessary that James give the command because the condition of the church (2:2-4) clearly indicated the prevalence of favoritism. Wealthy people were easily recognized and patronized with the best seats because they wore fine garments and gold rings on their fingers.

One might assume that the early church ushers were prejudiced. It would be much the same if ushers today seated the wealthy, the intelligent, the beautiful, and the popular in the most prominent seats in the sanctuary while disguising the less favorable. However, in God's eyes there are no distinctions. James 2:5-8 reminds us that God has chosen the poor in the eyes of the world to be rich in faith and to inherit the kingdom.

I will never forget a church usher named Paul Burkett that I met when I attended his church for the first Sunday I was away at college. As he stood at the entrance of the center aisle of the sanctuary, he smiled and grabbed my hand. I didn't have time to contemplate his missing fingers as his comments made me feel like I was the most important person to enter the sanctuary that day. Yet, he and I both must have known that I was just a "poor" college student who wouldn't be able to contribute much financially to that church. Needless to say, his church became mine during my college years and his home became a "home away from home" for me as well as countless others. He loved everyone and didn't show favoritism.

What would cause favoritism? There could be several causes. These early Christians could have been avoiding the issue of poverty, not wanting to face the responsibilities of helping the less fortunate. They may have wanted to be wealthy themselves, hoping to use the rich person as a means to that end. They could have been embarrassed for visitors to see the poor in the church. They could have assumed wrongly that the rich are the most blessed by God.

Whatever the cause, the condition was sinful (2:9) and needed to be cured. For the cure James tells us to obey the law (2:8-10) and understand its judgment (2:13). To show favoritism is to disobey the law. James reiterates the royal law, "Love your neighbor as yourself" and goes on to say that "if you show favoritism, you sin and are convicted by the law as lawbreakers . . . judgment without mercy will be shown to anyone who has not been merciful" (2:9, 13).

The best cure for showing favoritism is alluded to in 2:1. We are to look to Jesus as our example. If we look to Jesus, we will *see others as Jesus saw them*. First Samuel 16:7 says, "Man looks at the outward appearance, but the Lord looks at the heart." Jesus looks beyond the surface to the substance of a person. He sees beyond the problems to the potential. He saw "shifting sand" Peter as a potential rock (John 1:42). He saw the sinful Samaritan woman as a powerful witness in her community (John 4:39). We need to see others as Jesus sees them.

I'm reminded of walking along the beach with my younger daughter Kara one summer as she picked up shells. As I started to point out the ugliness of some broken shells, I suddenly stopped. "Oh, Mommy, isn't this one beautiful? I really like it. I want to keep this one." As her bucket filled, I thought about her nondiscriminating nature and about how Jesus must pick us up and love us in spite of our brokenness and ugliness.

If we look to Jesus as the example, we will also *feel with others as Jesus felt*. Isaiah 53:1-3 helps us realize the rejection that Jesus experienced. He understood and empathized with the rejected. Have you ever felt rejection? I have and it hurts. Yet, if we love as Jesus loved, we will not retaliate but use our understanding of rejection to minister to the hurting.

Have you ever watched or agonized over exercise videos or aerobic television programs. Now, we even have "Christian" exercise tapes. The variety is endless. I have a hard time watching and listening to the skinny person who never had to fight the battle of the bulge or overcome the temptation of treats. For her or him, "slim and trim" is easy and natural. However, I can truly tolerate—even get excited about the saint who strains, the one who understands, the one who has been where I've been; the one who honestly admits that double-stuffed Oreos are a temptation; the one who admits that exercise isn't like a stroll through the park with your loved one on a moonlit night.

I guess that is why I'm comforted when I read that God is our judge and that He will judge fairly (James 2:1-13). We are not to be respecters of persons. Just as Jesus sets the example for not showing favoritism, He also knows what it is like to be tempted. "For we do not have a high priest who is unable to sympathize with our weaknesses, but we have one who has been tempted in every way, just as we are—yet was without sin. Let us then approach the throne of grace with confidence, so that we may receive mercy and find grace to help us in our time of need" (Hebrews 4:15-16). The Lord is our spiritual fitness expert and only He has the right to judge and the ability to help us not judge others.

DISCIPLINING FOR
🍂 DAILY EXERCISE 🍂

SUNDAY: Approaching God's Word: 2 Corinthians 5:6-10
Applying God's Word:

Memorizing God's Word: Romans 14:11-12

MONDAY   Approaching God's Word: Proverbs 8:17-21
Applying God's Word:

TUESDAY: Approaching God's Word: Matthew 5:1-12
Applying God's Word:

WEDNESDAY: Approaching God's Word: Romans 13:8-10
Applying God's Word:

THURSDAY: Approaching God's Word: Matthew 22:37-40
Applying God's Word:

FRIDAY: Approaching God's Word: Ephesians 5:1-2
                           Applying God's Word:

SATURDAY: Approaching God's Word: Micah 6:6-8
                           Applying God's Word:

CHAPTER FIVE

THE

Tongue Tying

STRETCHING YOUR
♞ SPIRITUAL MUSCLES ♞

Read James 3:1-12.

1. Why is teaching the Word of God a serious matter? See also Hebrews 13:17. How might we encourage teachers?

2. Who is a "perfect" man according to James 3:2? Read Matthew 5:48. What do you think Jesus meant by "Be perfect"? Can a person be "perfect"? What do the following passages have to say about perfection?

Matthew 19:21

Colossians 3:14

1 Peter 4:8

1 John 3:2-3

3. What relationship does the tongue have to the whole body? How is the tongue described in James 3:3-5?

Give a one- or two-word description for this kind of tongue?

4. Give a one- or two-word description for the kind of tongue described in James 3:6.

5. Give a one- or two-word description for the kind of tongue described in James 3:9-12.

6. Complete the following chart on the positive and negative influences of the tongue.

	Positive Influence	Negative Influence
Proverbs 10:21		
Proverbs 11:9		
Proverbs 12:6		
Proverbs 12:18		
Proverbs 13:3		
Proverbs 15:1		
Proverbs 15:4		
Proverbs 16:21		
Proverbs 16:27		
Proverbs 18:21		

Think of a time when someone's tongue influenced you positive-ly—negatively. When was the last time you influenced someone with your tongue positively?—negatively?

7. What is the problem stated in James 3:7-8? According to the following Scriptures, what truly controls the tongue?

Matthew 12:34

Matthew 15:18-19

Proverbs 16:23

8. How will we be accountable for our tongues according to Matthew 12:36-37?

9. How can the following passages relate to taming the tongue?

Philippians 2:13, 4:8-9, 13

Colossians 3:15-17

Read James 3:13-18.
10. Contrast earthly and heavenly wisdom. How can earthly or heavenly wisdom affect the tongue?

11. Describe wisdom according to the following Scriptures:

Job 28:28

Proverbs 9:10

Matthew 7:24-25

Colossians 2:2-3

12. Who gives true heavenly wisdom? Check out Proverbs 2:6-8 and James 1:5-6.

What wisdom have you been seeking lately?

EXERCISING YOUR
❧ SPIRITUAL MUSCLES ❧

"I wish you were dead!" Hours later as I awakened to the flashing red light spiraling across my bedroom ceiling and walls, the words I had so flippantly spoken to my brother in a selfish moment of anger haunted the very depths of my saddened soul.

"Is it too late, Lord?—too late to tell him I'm sorry?—too late to tell him I love him?—too late to undo what I've done with my tongue?"

How often have you asked yourself, "Is it too late?" only to realize that, perhaps it is. Fortunately, for me on that New Year's Eve it wasn't. But I would never want to experience another six hours of waiting and wrestling like those again.

As my older brother Ron and I had practiced our accordion duet for the New Year's Watch Night Service at church, we began to argue over who would play what part. In the heat of the argument, I shouted the words which would later haunt me, "I wish you were dead!" We played perfectly and harmoniously for the people; not so harmoniously for ourselves and the Lord.

After taking his girlfriend home, he fell asleep and hit a tree a half mile from home. As I watched the ambulance crew load his battered and unconscious form, I cried to God for his life and my sanity. Two days later his smile greeted me as I tearfully lipped the words, "I love you!"

It seems strange that an incident which happened over 20 years ago still tempers and ties my tongue today. I learned the hard way how our tongues can so negatively trip us. James describes three tongues which have negative effects. I call them the "tongue trippers."

The first tongue described in James 3:3-5 is the *influential tongue.* Though the tongue is a small body part, it can wield powerful influence both negatively and positively. It is compared in this part of James to a horse's bit which controls the whole horse or a ship's rudder which directs the whole ship. In Proverbs we are told that the tongue has the power to destroy or give life; to bring healing or crush the spirit; to pierce like a sword or promote instruction. The tongue is virtually the fulcrum of a teeter-totter weighing down or lifting up a person. It all depends where the fulcrum is placed and how it is used.

I recall one spring when a former neighbor emerged from her home like a spring daffodil opening its petals to all who would observe. As I pushed my younger daughter Kara in the stroller, I began praising my neighbor for her obvious weight loss during the winter months. At which time, her husband chimed in with his cutting remarks, "No matter how hard she tries, she'll always be *behind* in her meals," while pointing to her behind. He loudly laughed while she silently cried. Needless to say, within a few weeks she had begun to put back on the weight. One slip of the husband's tongue had defeated months of hard work and discipline.

The second tongue James describes in James 3:5-6 is the *igniting tongue*. It is compared to a small spark which sets the whole forest ablaze. One false rumor can do untold damage. And once it starts, it is as hard to put out as an uncontrollable forest fire, blown and scattered to throw other sparks on otherwise calm scenes. We've all seen reputations ruined by a slight slip of the tongue. We can all be spiritual fire fighters by following a few rules of fire safety:

1. Avoid the flame. Avoid a gossip. (Proverbs 20:19; 1 Thessalonians 5:22)
2. Don't fan the flame. Do not share in the sins of others and do not encourage a gossip by listening. (1 Timothy 5:22)
3. Douse the flame. Confront and restore the gossip in the spirit of meekness. (Galatians 6:1-2)
4. Ask for a fire fighter's wisdom. Be a peacemaker. (James 1:5-7; 3:17-18)
5. Pray about the burns. (Philippians 4:6-7; 1 Peter 5:7)

The *inconsistent tongue* is the third tongue James describes in James 3:9-12. We all know someone whose tongue drips with sugar one moment and poison the next. Forced to walk on eggshells, we tiptoe circumspectly with fear and trepidation every moment we are in contact with the person. Usually people with inconsistent tongues struggle inwardly but outwardly never admit their struggles. James compares the inconsistent tongue to a spring that yields both fresh and salt water; to a fig tree that bears both figs and olives; to a grapevine that bears both grapes and figs. The inconsistent tongue deceives as well as destroys.

Unfortunately, we all can recall times when our tongues have tripped us. We identify so readily with James when he writes in 3:7 that "no man can tame the tongue." We say, "What's the use of even trying?"

No man can tame the tongue, but the Word of God encourages us to recognize that the Holy Spirit can transform and tie the tongue. Equal time must be given to the tongue "tiers" as well as "trippers."

To tie the tongue, one must, first of all, *check the condition of the heart.* The tongue is the temperature gauge on the heart's engine. If the engine overheats, then the temperature gauge warns us of engine trouble. If the tongue gets out of control, it is a sure sign that we need to check our heart. Matthew tells us that "a man's heart determines his speech. A good man's speech reveals the rich treasures within him. An evil-hearted man is filled with venom, and his speech reveals it" (Matthew 12:34-35, TLB). What does your tongue reveal about your heart? We need to constantly fill the heart with good things from God's Word in order to tie our tongues.

One must also *concede to the Spirit's control* to tie the tongue successfully. It always interested me that when James describes the tongue as a horse's bit that controls the horse or a ship's rudder that directs the ship, he, perhaps purposefully, fails to mention that a horse's bit must, in reality, be controlled by the rider and the ship's rudder must be controlled by the helmsman. I daily remind myself that the Lord, through the Holy Spirit, must be the rider or the helmsman controlling my tongue. Who is your helmsman?

If you have difficulty yielding control to the Lord, ask Him for the desire to give Him control. Philippians 2:13 states that "it is God who works in us both *to will* and *to act* according to His good purpose." When you have the willingness to concede control of your tongue, you'll soon discover you also have the strength to do it as well. Take a step at a time. Ask for His control of your tongue for a half hour; then an hour; then a day; then a week or more!

Interestingly enough, we have to constantly concede. I'm right now struggling with wanting to give my opinion to two, older, cranky couples sitting next to me at the swimming pool. They are cursing and complaining about the children in the pool, two of whom are mine. "O, Lord, help me!" I'm reminded of a miserable New Year's Eve over 20 years ago.

DISCIPLINING FOR
❦ DAILY EXERCISE ❦

SUNDAY: Approaching God's Word: Proverbs 18:13; 29:20
               Applying God's Word:

               Memorizing God's Word: Colossians 3:16-17

MONDAY: Approaching God's Word: Proverbs 10:19
               Applying God's Word:

TUESDAY: Approaching God's Word: Proverbs 26:28; 28:23;
               29:5
               Applying God's Word:

WEDNESDAY: Approaching God's Word: Proverbs 27:1-2
               Applying God's Word:

THURSDAY: Approaching God's Word: Proverbs 11:13; 17:9;
               18:8; 25:18
               Applying God's Word:

54

FRIDAY: Approaching God's Word: Proverbs 13:3; 21:23; 16:23-24; 15:23
Applying God's Word:

SATURDAY: Approaching God's Word: Philippians 4:8-9
Applying God's Word:

CHAPTER SIX

THE WHIRLPOOL OF

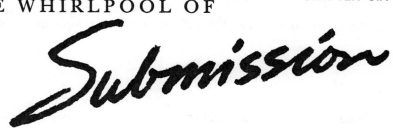

STRETCHING YOUR
&❧ SPIRITUAL MUSCLES &❧

Read James 4:1-17.

1. What causes conflicts among people?

How can "battles within" a person cause "battles without" in relationships with others?

2. What thoughts did Paul share in Romans 7:21–8:2 concerning his "battles within"?

What "battles within" are you waging? What comfort do you find in the words of Paul and James?

55

3. What reason in James 4:3 is given as to why people do not receive?

What motivates your prayers?

4. Why did James call the people "adulterous"? (4:4)

What does he mean by "friendship with the world"?

What do the following have to say regarding the results of friendship with the world?

	Examples of Friendship with World	Results
Matthew 6:24		
Matthew 13:22		
Matthew 16:26		

Examples of Friendship with World   Results

1 John 2:15-17

1 Timothy 6:10

Psalm 78:56-59

5. How can God be jealous? See also Exodus 34:14.

6. With what attitude can we better receive God's grace? How does
   God respond to the proud?

   Psalm 18:27   Proverbs 16:18
   Psalm 138:6   Isaiah 57:15
   Proverbs 3:34

7. What steps should we take to humble ourselves according to James
   4:7-10? What are the results?

   In what areas of your life have you been self-sufficient, not wanting
   the Lord's help? Are you willing to submit these to Him?

8. What do you think it means to "draw nigh to God"? What are the results? See also John 15:5-7 and Psalm 73:28.

9. With what is life compared? (James 2:14)

What are some other comparisons found in Scripture?

1 Chronicles 29:15   Psalm 103:15

Job 7:6   Isaiah 38:12

Job 9:25   1 Peter 1:24

Psalm 39:5

How, then, should we set our goals and make our plans?

Is there any good that you have procrastinated in doing? What are you going to do about it?

EXERCISING YOUR 🌿 *SPIRITUAL MUSCLES* 🌿

Have you ever received a gift you weren't too enthused about? I still recall my husband's words as he grinned excitedly. "Honey, I received a free membership for you to the local health spa tonight when I joined."

I'd really never thought of going to a health spa. After all, I had assumed that eight years of cheerleading couldn't have been so far removed that I would be that much out of shape. However, after my first visit to the spa, I realized that assuming was a mistake. Staying in shape needs to be a constant goal.

I remember the instructor carefully showing me the whirlpool. As she told me that I needed to climb in the whirlpool after exercising to help the sore muscles, I laughed to myself. I silently rebelled, *That sure looks hot and miserable to me. No way! I'm skipping this!*

As I awakened the next morning, every aching muscle in my body was shouting to me that I should have crawled into the whirlpool after exercising. I was paying for not submitting to the instructor's directions.

As the aches and pains of physical exercise can be soothed away in the spa's whirlpool, so spiritual aches and pains can be soothed away in God's whirlpool of submission. But we must submit to Him. We must not laughingly rebel by thinking, *No way. I don't need God. After all, I can handle this all by myself.*

James 4:1-17 has much to say about humbling ourselves and submitting to God. A closer look at James 4:1-7 will help us *realize our spiritual aches and pains;* tell us how to *rid ourselves of those aches and pains in God's whirlpool of submission;* and give us the inevitable *results of submission.*

Before I would ever have submitted to the heat and humidity of the spa's whirlpool, I had to realize the aches and pains as a result of not submitting to it. Before I would ever have submitted my will to God, I had to realize my own inadequacy and spiritual poverty. "Only when a man realizes his own ignorance can he ask the guidance of God. Only when a man realizes his own poverty in the things that matter will he pray for the riches of God's grace. Only when a man realizes his weakness in necessary things will he come to draw upon the strength of God. Only when a man realizes that he cannot cope with life by himself will he kneel before the Lord of all good life. Only when a man realizes his own sin will he realize his need of a Saviour and of the forgiveness of God" (William Barclay, *The Letters of James and Peter* [Philadelphia: Westminster Press, 1960], 129).

One can realize the spiritual aches and pains indicated by battles without and battles within. The battles without are fights and quarrels usually rooted in spiritual struggles and battles within a person. The biggest battle that James refers to in 4:4-5 is spiritual adultery. Now, why would James call the addressees adulterous? Romans 8:7-8 tells us that the sinful mind is hostile to God and does not submit to God's law. It is as wrong to have divided loyalties in our spiritual conditions as it is to have divided loyalties in a marriage relationship. God is a jealous God (Exodus 20:5; Deuteronomy 32:16; Matthew 6:24) and He wants our total allegiance. Just as there are checklists to help us avoid marital adultery, there are questions we can ask ourselves to avoid spiritual adultery such as: How much quality time do I spend with God? How consistently do I spend time with God? Am I enjoying the world's enticements? Is there anything or anyone that is more important to me than my relationship to Christ?

What if I told my husband, "I'm sorry. My life is so full right now with busy schedules and squeezed itineraries that two minutes next week and three hours next month is all I have time for you"? Or what if I said, "I'm sorry, but Joe Blow or Curly Cool seems much more interesting and, after all, my job is far more important than you"? What would happen to my marriage? Yet, many of us are giving similar excuses while neglecting the most important relationship of all—the one with the Lord Jesus Christ. We are committing spiritual adultery.

James 4:7-9 gives a progression of steps that must be taken to rid ourselves of spiritual aches and pains. Listed in order they are: submit to God (4:7); resist the Devil (4:7); draw near to God (4:8); cleanse our hands (4:8); purify our hearts (4:8); and be sorrowfully repentant (4:9).

When we humble ourselves before God, we admit that our worth comes from Him alone. We have done nothing to deserve His grace and favor (Romans 3:23), yet He loves us and gives us value and dignity. "For we are God's workmanship created in Christ Jesus to do good works, which God prepared in advance for us to do" (Ephesians 2:10). But before we can do His good works, our hearts must be pure. We must humbly confess our sins. We must realize our sufficiency comes from Him. Just as a cracked vase is useless to hold water for flowers, God cannot use a prideful person to show forth His glory.

God does not ask of us anything that He himself has not experienced. Read Philippians 2:5-11 to understand how Jesus set the supreme example of submission as He humbled himself to become a man and obey His Father all the way to the Cross.

The results of getting rid of our spiritual aches and pains in God's whirlpool of submission are grace, strength, and peace. James 4:1-3 says it is difficult to receive peace when you ask with wrong motives. James 4:6 says, "He gives grace to the humble," and 4:10 says, "He will lift you up."

An old fable passed down through the years tells of a beggar who sat beside the road collecting rice grains in his bowl as the villagers thronged the narrow streets to catch a glimpse of the royal prince as he would soon pass through their area.

As the prince approached, he noticed the lonely beggar and motioned his chariot driver to stop. He quietly asked the beggar for the rice grains in his bowl. Now, if I'd been the beggar, I would have probably protested, thinking that the prince had all he wanted. Why would he want or even need my only means of livelihood—a few measly rice grains? What would you have done? The beggar, however, submissively gave his rice grains to the prince.

It is at this point that I might start feeling sorry for the beggar. But as the prince pulled away, the beggar glanced into his bowl. For every rice grain the prince had taken, he had put a ruby in its place. Submission had its rewards for the beggar and submission has its rewards for us.

DISCIPLINING FOR
🎵 DAILY EXERCISE 🎵

SUNDAY: Approaching God's Word: 2 Chronicles 7:14
       Applying God's Word:

       Memorizing God's Word: James 4:6-7

MONDAY: Approaching God's Word: Psalm 25:9
       Applying God's Word:

TUESDAY: Approaching God's Word: Psalm 149:4
       Applying God's Word:

WEDNESDAY: Approaching God's Word: Matthew 23:12
       Applying God's Word:

THURSDAY: Approaching God's Word: Luke 14:11; Romans
       12:3
       Applying God's Word:

FRIDAY: Approaching God's Word: 1 Peter 5:5-6
                    Applying God's Word:

SATURDAY: Approaching God's Word: Philippians 2:5-8
                    Applying God's Word:

CHAPTER SEVEN

THE PREVENTATIVE

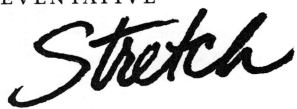

STRETCHING YOUR
🕊 *SPIRITUAL MUSCLES* 🕊

Read James 5:1-6.

1. What have the godless rich done with their riches? What have the riches done to the godless rich?

2. According to Matthew 6:19-20, where are we encouraged to attain riches?

3. What is considered great gain in 1 Timothy 6:6? Can you think of a specific time in your life when you didn't have much materially but were perfectly content and happy?

4. According to 1 Timothy 6:17-19, what are the wealthy to do with their money? What then should be our motivation if we want to get rich? Do you hold tightly or loosely to your possessions and money?

Read James 5:7-18.

5. With what does James compare waiting for the Lord's return?

6. How do we know the Lord will return? Examine Acts 1:11 and Hebrews 9:28.

When will He return? Check out Matthew 24:27, 36 and Luke 12:10.

7. Who are good examples in the face of suffering? Why?

What comfort is found in James 5:11 for those who suffer? From our accumulative studies in James, how would you counsel a friend in the midst of suffering?

8. Read 2 Corinthians 12:7-10. If God doesn't deliver from suffering, what does He do? Relate an incident in your life or another's when God's grace was sufficient.

9. How does James say we should react when we are happy? When is the last time you truly reacted this way? Read Psalms 103–104 to help you in your reactions.

10. What should be done for the sick?

   How would you describe the prayer of faith? See also 1 John 5:14-15.

   Does God always heal as a result of prayer? How is Romans 8:26 comforting when we don't know how to pray for the sick?

11. Much emphasis is given to prayer in the book of James. Tradition tells us that James practiced what he preached. He spent so much time on his knees in prayer that his knees were tough and enlarged. Thus, he was called "Camel Knees." If someone were to nickname you according to your prayer life, what would it be? What would you like it to be?

12. Read 1 Kings 16:29–17:6. Why did Elijah, the praying prophet, pray that God would withhold rain from Israel?

Write how God has answered a specific prayer for you this past year?

For what have you earnestly and fervently prayed more recently?

EXERCISING YOUR
❧ SPIRITUAL MUSCLES ❧

Thirteen miles was my goal! A couple of years ago I trained with my friend, Shelly, to run the Indianapolis Mini-Marathon, an annual run which takes place two days before the Indianapolis 500 race. The exhilarating marathon starts at the circle in downtown Indy and ends at the finish line of the 500 Track.

A big part of the training program was the warm-up of stretching my body muscles to prevent injuries and soreness during and after the running. Interestingly enough, no matter how far I would run, one mile or seven, I would do the same stretching exercises. They are as necessary as proper running shoes. They serve as prevention from injuries as well as preparation for a good run.

In the spiritual realm, there must be preventative and preparatory stretching as well. The injuries from lack of spiritual stretching are experiencing the *futility of riches* and missing the *richness of the future*.

James addresses the futility of riches in 5:1-6 when he describes how riches fail (vv. 1-3), rob (v. 4), and kill (vv. 5-6). He is not condemning riches—rather the attitude of living only and primarily for riches. In New Testament times a man was considered wealthy by his amassing of grain, garments, and gold or silver. Yet, the futility lay in the fact that in the end the grain became rotten, the garments riddled, and the gold rusted. Have you seen any storage sheds beside grave markers in the cemeteries lately? The amassing of wealth today is just as futile as it was in biblical times. The media constantly bombarding us with the "I want" and "you need" messages makes it easy for us to be sucked into the empty vacuum of worldly nothingness.

In contrast to the futility of riches, James pictures the richness of the future—the Lord's Coming. We must not miss the richness of the future with the Lord eternally because of the futility of riches momentarily.

James 5:7-18 contains three components of the preventative stretch, what we must do to be prepared for the Lord's coming. James 5:7 encourages us to *be patient*, even in the midst of suffering. Our patience is to be compared to the farmer waiting patiently for his planted crop to come to fruition. The Greek word for patience is *hupomone* which describes that which holds on steadfastly in spite. In spite of what? In spite of suffering, injustice, and disappointments.

I often laugh at the impatience I felt when pregnant with our first child. I'm sure other expectant parents must experience impatience as well. The pregnancy was rough and I even spent time in the hospital at the point of dehydration. I thought it would never end. However, nothing I could do would have caused an earlier arrival. In fact, Kim came three weeks late, weighing in at nine and a half pounds. The minute we saw her, we knew she was worth the wait. And the moment our eyes meet the Lord's, He will immediately dispel any thought that it wasn't worth the wait.

Secondly, James tells us to *be on patrol*. Just as the farmer watches for his crops to mature while protecting and nurturing them, we need to be living every moment as if Jesus would come that very moment. First John 2:28 refers to being on patrol as "continuing in Him, so that when He appears we may be confident and unashamed before Him at His coming."

I love the story from Nehemiah which describes how the Israelites posted a guard to patrol for the enemies while they completed the wall. Being on patrol involves always looking while always learning and living.

Lastly, we are commanded to *be prayerful* in trouble and triumph (James 5:13). Prayer is a tremendous privilege we often take for granted. While traveling with my husband who was preaching throughout the British Isles for OMS International, I spent an exhilarating and exhausting first night at the mission headquarters in Manchester, England. A twenty-two-year-old Japanese girl named Emiko came to the home and introduced herself as a Christian who had come to England to learn English. After tea (or supper for Americans), we engaged in conversation. There were two things I thought we had in common—a deep love for the Lord and a deep interest in English. I had taught high school English and journalism and thought I could help some before she started her classes. Yet, little did I know, when our conversation began, that her greatest need was not to learn English but to know who Jesus was and how He died for her. Not long into the conversation, I detected she knew very little of Christ, let alone Christianity. Her definition of being a Christian was, "I'm not Communist; but I do want to know about Jesus."

Have you ever tried to introduce someone to Jesus Christ whose language you did not know and who knew little of your language? Interesting predicament! Yet, God was gracious. With flannelgraph in hand and prayer in my heart, I began. The Spirit obviously opened her eyes and heart, and before our evening was over, Emiko, a Japanese Buddhist, had accepted Christ as her Saviour.

After six weeks of discipling, we met together for the last time. Tearfully, I asked if she had any difficulties or questions. "Yes, I have trouble praying," she said.

After further questioning, I realized her difficulty lay in the fact that she thought God only understood English. When I told her He understood all languages, including Japanese, she beamed, "No problem! No problem!"

Oh, how we limit God. Oh, how we forget what a privilege it is to pray to Him.

Prayer must be a *priority*, yet how often do we pray as a last resort? I was once challenged by a devotional for women I read in *Good Morning Lord* (Baker Books) which told of an African village whose first Christians responded to the necessity of making their time with God a priority. They each chose a tree in the jungle and, as time passed, wore a path to each tree. The paths were called God-paths. I was forced to ask myself, "If someone would see my God-path in the jungle growth, would it be clearly defined from wear, or would it be overgrown and hardly noticeable due to neglect?" What about your God-path? First Thessalonians 5:17 challenges us to pray continually.

Prayer is a *peace giver*. James 5:13 says if we're in trouble, we should pray. God doesn't always change the circumstances but can give calmness in the midst of them. We all can attest to times of trial when God took our hand and guided us. He's done so for me innumerable times. I've often heard people say, "If someone had told me I would be in these circumstances years, weeks, or even days before, I would have said I couldn't have coped. Yet, God is sufficient!" He only gives the grace when it is needed.

I remember a time when His strength was there when I needed it. I cried for God to help as my eyes glanced into the rear-view mirror of my little Volkswagen while trying to turn into the high school where I taught. I knew the semi-truck was approaching too rapidly to stop in time. As my body endured the grueling turmoil and pain, my soul experienced God's presence and peace in indescribable ways. His peace was mine because I had cried out to Him. His peace can be yours in any situation. Just ask.

Lastly, prevailing prayer can be a real *power source*. James 5:17-18 reminds us of Elijah who earnestly prayed for the rain to stop and start again after three and a half years. Now that's powerful praying! When was the last time you saw a seemingly impossible situation turned around because of prayer? Many times patience must parallel the prayer. After several months of praying, we recently saw a hopeless situation turn around for a close friend in our support group. Even if the situation had not turned around, we have seen the power of prayer as the Lord uplifted her and gave her strength for every moment of the difficult time.

One of the most powerful demonstrations of prayer I've ever heard of was the winter the river didn't freeze. It was a winter in the early seventies that South Korean Christians prayed earnestly that the Imjin River dividing South Korea from communist North Korea would not freeze. After hearing of rumors that the North Korean ruler felt it was his best astrological year to invade and capture South Korea by driving tanks across the river when it froze, the Christians made the situation a top priority in prayer.

Realizing the threat to their freedom of religion, they entreated the Lord at their early morning prayer meetings. Yes, at 5:00 every morning Korean Christians still meet for prayer. I wouldn't have believed it if I had not seen it for myself while visiting missionary friends in Korea. They also proclaimed days of fasting and prayer. Could God not answer such an earnest and honest request? It was one of the mildest winters in Korean history and the Imjin River never froze.

When writing about prayer, James was writing about something he had experienced. Tradition indicates that because of the many hours he spent on his knees in prayer, his friends nicknamed him "Camel Knees." If you were given a nickname for your prayer life, what would it be? Could it be "Stretch" because you consider being in prayer, being patient, and being on patrol just as important and vital as a runner considers stretching while training to run a marathon?

DISCIPLINING FOR
🎵 DAILY EXERCISE 🎵

SUNDAY: Approaching God's Word: Mark 1:35; Luke 6:12-13
Applying God's Word:

Memorizing God's Word: Philippians 4:6-7

MONDAY: Approaching God's Word: Matthew 7:7-11
Applying God's Word:

TUESDAY: Approaching God's Word: Luke 11:1-13
Applying God's Word:

WEDNESDAY: Approaching God's Word: Acts 4:25-31
Applying God's Word:

THURSDAY: Approaching God's Word: 1 Timothy 2:1-8
Applying God's Word:

FRIDAY: Approaching God's Word: 1 John 5:14-15
Applying God's Word:

SATURDAY: Approaching God's Word: Colossians 1:9-14
Applying God's Word:

CHAPTER EIGHT

THE SPIRITUAL

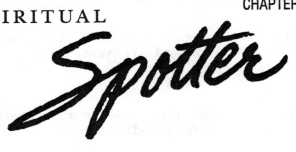

STRETCHING YOUR
✿ SPIRITUAL MUSCLES ✿

Read James 5:19-20.
1. What does James challenge Christians to do?

2. What is the Truth?

According to the following Scriptures, how must a person react to Truth?

Galatians 5:7

2 Corinthians 4:2

2 Thessalonians 2:10

1 John 3:19

3. What can Truth do for a person? How? (John 8:32)

4. How do we understand the Truth? (John 16:12-15)

Describe a time when this happened to you.

5. What do you think causes a person to wander from the Truth?

What caused Demas, who had been a faithful follower of Paul's (Colossians 4:14, Philemon 24) to wander? (2 Timothy 4:9-10)

What things cause you to wander from the Truth?

6. What will result if someone helps turn a sinner from his errors?

7. Do you think it is easy or comfortable to confront a person who has wandered from the Truth? Why or why not?

Have you ever been the confronter or the recipient of a confrontation concerning spiritual wandering? How did you feel?

8. According to Matthew 18:15-18, how are we to confront?

If the other person won't listen, then what steps should be taken?

9. With what attitude should we always confront? (Galatians 6:1-2)

10. According to Matthew 7:1-5, what must we first do before we can point out flaws in others? Does this passage give permission to confront another?

EXERCISING YOUR
⁂ SPIRITUAL MUSCLES ⁂

After wandering through the deep woods for over an hour and a half, the little girl squeezing my sweaty palm meekly inquired, "Miss Vicki, are we possibly lost?"

In my heart I knew we were lost, but how could I tell 15 little girls who trusted me as their junior counselor that I had gone astray? At that moment I suddenly saw a familiar sight, a large, gnarled tree in a clearing approximately 50 yards ahead.

"No, sweetheart, we're not lost. We've just wandered from the path a little. We'll be back at our cabin in about 20 minutes and I know Miss Coretta will be so glad to see us," I calmly reassured her and myself.

I was right! Coretta, my head counselor, as well as the rest of the staff of Camp Berean, were all glad to see us. Coretta lovingly asked, "What happened? Where have you been?"

I quickly replied, "I wish I knew! We must have strayed from the path just enough to get turned around. I wish you'd been along. You know the path so much better than I and you wouldn't have let me wander."

Wouldn't it be great if there were people in our lives at all times to keep us from going off the spiritual path of life—to keep us accountable for staying spiritually fit? Instead of Weight Watchers we'd have Spiritual Spotters.

I have watched both my daughters at gymnastics lessons and am always more relieved when I see the teacher "spotting" the girls on the gymnastics apparatus. *Webster's Dictionary* defines a spotter as one who locates enemy hazards and targets. When my daughters' teacher is spotting, she is looking out for any possible falls or injuries and is in a position to physically prevent them.

In the book of Nehemiah, the Jews "posted a guard" for each other as some would work at rebuilding the wall and some would watch for the enemies. Likewise, we should serve as Spiritual Spotters for one another, willing to post a guard at all times. The last two verses of James recognize the importance of spiritual spotting for one another.

First of all, James addresses the *situation* of the spiritual wanderer. Secondly, he acknowledges a *solution*—the value of a restorer, the spiritual spotter.

In 5:19 when James writes about the wanderer, he is clearly referring to the believer who has fallen into sin and is no longer living a consistent life. He or she has neglected the reality and relevance of Truth, God's Word. James clearly indicates that the wanderer is in serious danger and needs to be confronted and restored.

Wandering is also a dangerous position because the wanderer can lead others astray, much like I was responsible for the 15 little girls losing their way in the woods. Many parents who willfully wander from the truth of God's Word and neglect the Lord and the church live to see their lack of spiritual fitness reaped in the lives of their children. "If only I had . . ." joins the list of life's most regretful phrases.

The solution for the wanderer is confrontation by a believer who truly cares about the wanderer and is willing to serve as spiritual spotter. James 5:19 says the spotter will help the wanderer understand the Word. "He should bring him back" and "save him from death and cover many sins."

Galatians 6:1-2 and Matthew 18:15-18 could serve as a good commentary of James 5:19-20. From these combined passages one could readily comprise a checklist for the Spiritual Spotter.

1. Do you have an established trust with the wanderer?
2. Have you prayed about your involvement in the restoration?
3. What are your motivations? Why are you confronting? Is your own ego intact? Are you wanting to retaliate?
4. Will you confront immediately and properly according to Matthew 18?
5. Will you insure confidentiality?
6. Can you confirm your accusations accurately?
7. Will you give constructive not destructive criticism?
8. Will you make yourself available to help the wanderer?

There are many who are walking the balance beam of spiritual fitness depending upon us to be their spiritual spotters. I want to meet the challenge. I want others to spot for me as well. How about you?

DISCIPLINING FOR
❧ DAILY EXERCISE ❧

SUNDAY: Approaching God's Word: Proverbs 27:17
                Applying God's Word:

                Memorizing God's Word: Galatians 6:1-2

MONDAY: Approaching God's Word: 1 Corinthians 10:12
                Applying God's Word:

TUESDAY: Approaching God's Word: 1 Thessalonians 5:9-11, 14
                Applying God's Word:

WEDNESDAY: Approaching God's Word: 2 Thessalonians 3:13-16
                Applying God's Word:

THURSDAY: Approaching God's Word: 2 Timothy 2:24-26
                Applying God's Word:

FRIDAY: Approaching God's Word: Hebrews 10:24
       Applying God's Word:

SATURDAY: Approaching God's Word: Romans 1:11-12
       Applying God's Word:

❧ LEADER'S GUIDE 1 ❧

Objective
To encourage group members to trust the Lord in the trials of life.

Personal Preparation
☐ Complete the Stretching Your Spiritual Muscles section of chapter 1.
☐ Read the Exercising Your Spiritual Muscles section.
☐ Complete the Disciplining for Daily Exercise section.
☐ Secure the following to take to this session: an old pen or pencil which still writes, 3 x 5 cards, envelopes, and a small trash can.

Group Participation
☐ Ask: **Have any of you ever been sore after exercising? Why are you sore? What comfort do you find in the soreness?** State: **James is a book that encourages us to flex our spiritual muscles and exercise our flabby faith in order to become firm in our faith in the Lord Jesus Christ. Let us read James 1:1-12.** Have each person read a verse until finished.
☐ Have group members share the insights and examples from questions 1 and 2.
☐ Hold up the "imperfect" pen or pencil. State: **According to the meaning of perfection "telios" in James 1:4, this pen is perfect. Why do you think it is perfect?** (It is perfect because it can be perfectly used for what it is intended.) **Describe a person that God is using perfectly.**
☐ Ask: **If you could ask for anything, for what would you ask? It isn't always easy to ask, yet God tells us in James 1:5-6 that He will give us wisdom if we ask without doubting.**
☐ Have group members share their findings for question 5.
☐ Have group members respond to question 6.
☐ Divide the group into pairs. Challenge them to quote to one another the Scripture memory from Romans 8:28.
☐ Pass out 3 x 5 cards. Tell members to write down a specific trial that they are presently experiencing. After they are finished, give each person an envelope in which to place the card. Pray: **Lord, we bring our trials to You. Help us to release them to You and allow You to make us better—not bitter . . . victors—not victims. We ask for Your wisdom in dealing with our trials.** After the prayer, tell the members to tear up the envelopes and their contents as a symbol of releasing them to God.

❧ LEADER'S GUIDE 2 ❧

Objective

To encourage group members to realize not only the process of temptation but also the protection against it available in the Lord.

Personal Preparation

☐ Complete the Stretching Your Spiritual Muscles section of chapter 2.

☐ Read the Exercising Your Spiritual Muscles section.

☐ Complete the Disciplining for Daily Exercise section.

☐ Talk to a fisherman or read about the different kinds of bait and lures used to attract various fish.

☐ Secure a tackle box full of a variety of bait and lures. Place a label on the outside that says, "Satan's Tackle Box." You may want to place tags on the various lures that might read—"pride, gluttony, lust, greed, idolatry, selfishness, etc."

Group Participation

☐ Pull out the tackle box. State: **We are going to talk about the process of temptation and protection against it but, first of all, I thought you might like to take a peek into Satan's tackle box. These are baits and lures he dangles before you and me.** If you haven't tagged the lures, then distribute the lures to the group and ask each person to name the lure with a temptation Satan uses. Start the discussion by describing one lure.

☐ Have members share insights gained from question 1.

☐ Discuss question 3.

☐ Have members give their answers to question 5. Ask: **Which character trait of God is most important to you at this time in your life?**

☐ State: **We all read in Matthew 4 how Jesus used God's Word to combat Satan. Let's read the Hebrews 4:12 description of God's Word. Are there other ways you could describe God's Word? Could you share a time when God's Word was the weapon you used to overcome temptation?** Be prepared to share yourself.

☐ Divide the group into pairs. Challenge them to quote to one another the Scripture memory from 1 Corinthians 10:13.

☐ Close with prayer for one another to be strong in overcoming temptation. Some may want to share specific requests.

❧ *LEADER'S GUIDE 3* ❧

Objective

To encourage group members to show forth tangible evidence of their faith.

Personal Preparation

☐ Complete the Stretching Your Spiritual Muscles section of chapter 3.

☐ Read the Exercising Your Spiritual Muscles section.

☐ Complete the Disciplining for Daily Exercise section.

☐ Prepare a tray of soil (with stones, clumps of grass, and weeds) which needs to be prepared before seeds can be planted.

☐ Gather small garden tools and marigold or other seeds that will germinate within four weeks.

☐ If you are brave enough, don't brush your hair or improve your appearance before the lesson. Bring a mirror, brush, toothbrush, make-up, etc. to class.

Group Participation

☐ If you decided to come to this session without brushing your hair, start the class by looking into a mirror and saying, "Oh, excuse me, I looked into the mirror earlier but didn't do anything about my appearance. I'll try now to make myself presentable. Our lesson today in James says that reading God's Word and not doing anything about it is like looking into a mirror and not doing anything about our appearance. If you go to class already groomed, just hold up the mirror and ask, "Approximately how many times have you looked into a mirror today? Did you make any changes?" Read James 1:22-25. James says that reading God's Word is much like looking into a mirror. Have you made any changes after looking into God's Word?

☐ Have group members discuss their answers to question 1.

☐ Have group members relate their answers to question 3. Show the tray of soil. As you discuss the answers, pass the tray around and ask the group members to remove the rocks, pull the weeds, and break up the soil.

☐ Ask: **Could you describe a time when you were truly receptive to the Word of God in your life? Describe a time in your life when you weren't receptive to the Word of God. What hindered your receptivity?**

☐ Have group members discuss answers to question 8.

☐ Ask: **According to the passages we read and the questions we answered for the lesson in James, what should be the evidence of our faith?** Silently reflect: **If someone were trying you for your faith think of all the evidence that could be used against you.**

☐ Divide into pairs and have the members quote to one another the memory work from Ephesians 2:10.

☐ Pass around the tray of soil and ask each person to quickly plant a seed. As you sprinkle water on the surface, pray the following: **Lord, just as we've prepared this soil today to receive these seeds, help us prepare our own hearts to receive your Word. As we watch these seeds grow over the next few weeks, make us fruitful in our spiritual lives as well. We want our faith to be evidenced by our actions. Help us work out our faith so that others might know.**

❧ *LEADER'S GUIDE 4* ❧

Objective
To encourage group members to be impartial and not show favoritism in their relationships.

Personal Preparation
☐ Complete the Stretching Your Spiritual Muscles section of chapter 4.
☐ Read the Exercising Your Spiritual Muscles section.
☐ Complete the Disciplining for Daily Exercise section.
☐ Think of a time when you experienced rejection.
☐ Make a list of your acquaintances and friendships. Ask yourself if they come from all walks of life—poor, wealthy, educated, uneducated, beautiful, homely, sinners, saints, etc.
☐ Take blank paper for each member to class.

Group Participation
☐ Ask: **Have any of you ever experienced rejection? Would anyone be willing to share how it felt?** Be prepared to share yourself.
☐ Ask: **Why are people rejected?** Read Isaiah 53:3, 7 and 1 Peter 2:21-24. **How did Jesus experience rejection?**
☐ State: **If we love as Jesus loved, we won't retaliate for an injustice, but will see to it that others are not rejected and no favoritism is displayed.**
☐ Have members share insights gained from question 2 from the Stretching the Spiritual Muscles section.
☐ Have members share their responses gained from question 5.
☐ Give group members blank pieces of paper. Have them write down a list of approximately 10–15 acquaintances or friendships. As they peruse their lists, ask them if the listees represent all walks of life—poor, wealthy, educated, uneducated, beautiful, homely, etc. They don't need to respond verbally.
☐ Have members discuss their answers to the last half of question 6. Share the following prayer written by Mother Theresa:

> "Dearest Lord, May I see you today and everyday in the person of your sick, your poor, and whilst nursing them, minister to you. Though you hide yourself behind the unattractive disguise of the irritable, the exacting, may I still recognize

You and say 'Jesus, my patient, how sweet it is to be serving You.' " (*Virtue*, December 1984, p. 25)

☐ State: **We read in Romans 14:10-13 that God is to be our judge. Why is it comforting to know that He is our only "fitness expert"?**

☐ Divide the group into pairs. Challenge them to quote to one another the Scripture memory from Romans 14:11-12.

☐ Close with prayer for one another to not be respecters of persons but to love as Christ loves.

❧ LEADER'S GUIDE 5 ❧

Objective
To encourage group members to seek God's guidance and strength for controlling their tongues.

Personal Preparation
☐ Complete the Stretching Your Spiritual Muscles section of chapter 5.
☐ Read the Exercising Your Spiritual Muscles section.
☐ Complete the Disciplining for Daily Exercise section.
☐ Buy tongue depressors for each member of the group.

Group Participation
☐ Have a group member take a pinch of salt or sugar and throw it into the air. Then ask the person to please retrieve every bit of the substance. Impossible! (You may blow bubbles instead.) Use this opportunity to explain the impossibility of retrieving our words once they have been spoken. Ask: **Would someone be willing to share a time when you wished you could have retrieved some spoken words?** Be prepared to share yourself if no one shares.

☐ Have members share insights gained from question 6 from the Stretching the Spiritual Muscles section.

☐ Ask: **Why do you think it is so difficult to control your tongue? Someone else's tongue?**

☐ Have group members read Colossians 3:16-17 together. Ask: **What is the key to richly teaching and admonishing one another? How does one cultivate a grateful heart?**

☐ State that verse 17 is an extremely challenging accomplishment. It is one, however, we should all strive to accomplish.

☐ Give each group member a tongue depressor and allow time to write Colossians 3:17 on it. Tell them to use the depressor as a bookmark in their Bibles as a constant reminder of God's willingness to tie the tongue.

☐ Divide the group into pairs. Challenge them to quote to each other the Scripture memory from Colossians 3:16-17.

☐ Encourage group members to share their spiritual needs for tying their tongues. Close with prayer for the Lord's control over each other's tongues.

✦ *LEADER'S GUIDE 6* ✦

Objective
To encourage group members to have submissive attitudes in their relationships with the Lord, which results in submissive attitudes in all their relationships.

Personal Preparation
☐ Complete the Stretching Your Spiritual Muscles section of chapter 6.
☐ Read the Exercising Your Spiritual Muscles section.
☐ Complete the Disciplining for Daily Exercise section.
☐ Think of a time when you experienced peace as a result of submitting to God's will for you.
☐ Describe a person you know that exemplifies humility and submission.
☐ Secure a sample piece of corduroy, velvet, or carpet with a nap.

Group Participation
☐ Show the sample piece of corduroy, velvet, or carpet. Rub the material with the grain to show the beauty of the material. Then rub a spot against the grain to show how it mars the beauty of the fabric. State: **Today's passage, James 4:1-17, will show us how submission is in accordance with God's will and only enhances the beauty of our spiritual fitness when we are not going against the grain.**
☐ Ask: **What do you think "submission" means? Describe a person you know that exemplifies humility and submission.** Be prepared to share your own answer.
☐ Have members give the insights and results they gained from question 4.
☐ Ask: **How do you respond to a proud person? How does God respond to a prideful attitude?** You may refer to the Scriptures in question 6.
☐ Have members give the steps they answered in question 7. Ask: **Could you share with the group a time when you experienced peace as a result of submitting to God's will?** Be prepared to share.
☐ State: **From the scriptural references given in question 9 we realized the finiteness of this life. How did you feel as you read the verses? How should these thoughts affect our goals and future plans?**
☐ Divide the group into pairs. Challenge them to quote to one another the Scripture memory from James 4:6-7.

☐ Ask the group members to think of any areas of their lives they have not submitted to God. Read aloud the beggar story from Exercising the Spiritual Muscles. Pray for yourself and them to have a submissive spirit.

❦ LEADER'S GUIDE 7 ❦

Objective
To encourage group members to see the priority of being spiritually prepared for the richness of the future rather than being pulled by the futility of present riches.

Personal Preparation
☐ Complete the Stretching Your Spiritual Muscles section of chapter 7.
☐ Read the Exercising Your Spiritual Muscles section.
☐ Complete the Disciplining for Daily Exercise section.
☐ Write a list of all the reasons why you should pray?
☐ Create a drawing that depicts your "prayer life" journey through the years.
☐ Take blank paper to class for each group member.

Group Participation
☐ Ask: **What do you think makes a person truly content? Would you share a specific time when you didn't have much materially but were perfectly content and happy?**
☐ Ask: **If we are not rich materially, how could we share with others? How could we show contentment with what we have?**
☐ Have group members share insights gained from question 3. Have the group come up with a combined definition of contentment.
☐ State: **James talks of patience in suffering in 5:10-11 and gives Job as an example of one who stayed true in spite of suffering.** Read together 2 Corinthians 12:7-10 to see what God did for Paul even though He didn't take away his infirmity. Encourage group members to share a time when God's grace was sufficient for them or another person.
☐ Read James 5:16-17 together. Ask: **To what extent do you think we should confess our sins to one another? Why do you think it is important to confess our sins to one another?**
☐ Have group members share their responses to question 12. This should be a rich time of sharing as they tell of answered prayer.
☐ Have group members share one helpful hint that has encouraged or helped their prayer lives.
☐ Give the group members the blank pieces of paper and have them draw an illustration that has depicted their prayer journey through the years. They should also write goals for improvement in their

prayer lives. Encourage them to keep this in their Bible and pray about the improvement.

☐ Divide the group into pairs. Challenge them to quote to one another the Scripture memory from Philippians 4:6-7.

☐ Close with prayer for one another to be content with material possessions and challenged to develop a deeper prayer life.

❦ *LEADER'S GUIDE 8* ❦

Objective
To encourage group members to be willing to humbly and willingly confront spiritual wanderers, those who have strayed from the Truth.

Personal Preparation
- ☐ Complete the Stretching Your Spiritual Muscles section of chapter 8.
- ☐ Read the Exercising Your Spiritual Muscles section.
- ☐ Complete the Disciplining for Daily Exercise section.
- ☐ If possible, secure a picture or poster of someone "spotting" a gymnast. You may need to ask someone to draw a cartoon or picture for you.

Group Participation
- ☐ Ask: **Could any of you relate a time when you were lost? How did you get lost? What emotions did you experience?**
- ☐ Read James 5:19-20. State: **James is describing a believer who is wandering from the spiritual path and relating our responsibility to the wanderer. What is our responsibility?**
- ☐ Have group members relate their thoughts and answers to the first part of question 5 from Stretching the Spiritual Muscles.
- ☐ Have group members share their thoughts on question 7.
- ☐ Have someone read Galatians 6:1-2 and Matthew 18:15-18. Ask· **According to these verses how should we approach the wanderer?**
- ☐ Pose the following hypothetical situation: **Jane is a good friend of yours. In fact, Jane and you have been prayer partners for two years. Lately, you have noticed that Jane is missing your scheduled prayer times frequently and is attending church sporadically. Just yesterday you accidentally saw her holding hands with a man who isn't her husband at a restaurant on the other side of town. What should you do?**
- ☐ Hold up the picture of the "spotter" spotting the gymnast. State: **Picture yourself as the gymnast and think of a time when you were struggling on the balance beam of spiritual fitness. Could you share with the group who your spotter was and how he or she helped you?**
- ☐ State: **Picture yourself as the spotter for someone else on the balance beam of spiritual fitness. Answer silently the following questions: Who is the gymnast? Who are you helping spiritually to**

keep from wandering from the truth of God's Word?

□ Divide the group into pairs. Challenge them to quote to one another the Scripture memory from Galatians 6:1-2.

□ Close with prayer for one another to become true spiritual spotters